ON ANTI-PSYCHIATRY
A patient's view
Part One

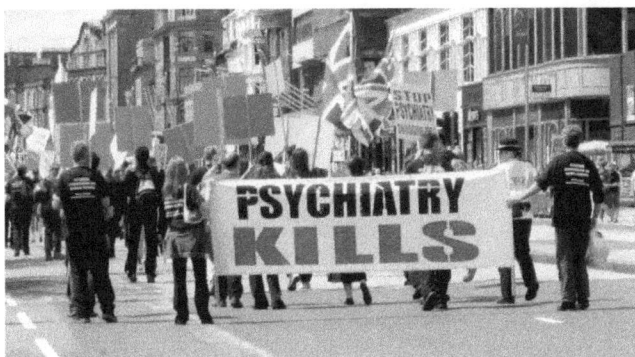

By Mark Ellerby

Mark Ellerby

Published by:
Chipmunkapublishing

www.chipmunkapublishing.com

Copyright © 2007 Mark Ellerby

Proofread by Ray Brazier

ON ANTI-PSYCHIATRY

The anti-psychiatry movement.

It is easy to some across the anti-psychiatry movement these days, especially where the family or patient has internet access. The views of Foucault and Goffman seem to paint the whole world of mental health in black.

I believe it is necessary to be more positive about the mental health system and for the social worker to receive training to explain the other side to the argument. I was left to figure it all out for myself that these views are not necessarily the only ones available.

Stigma is created in a capitalist society whose primary values are self reliance and self responsibility. In today's terms this is the equivalent of teaching independence and rehabilitation, especially through the policy of care in the community.

The great confinement of which Foucault wrote is therefore now over. The new issue is what is called under the latest terminology, 'social exclusion.' In actual fact the policy of community care allows many freedoms of the individual which was its intended basis.

We can choose our friends and relationships from the tremendous diversity of people at day centres. We have the financial freedom of controlling our own disability money and to live and go where we please. My personal view is that I can live quite happily and anonymously in this society taking advantage of these freedoms.

Crucially therefore, if other people want to think I am `mad' then that is up to them. If every body could adopt this attitude then stigma would matter much less than it does.

The anti-psychiatry movement nevertheless still attempts to exploit mental health for its own political ends. Any attempt to help people with mental illness is seen as a form of control of those who it holds to be alienated by a society where they cannot be so self-reliant.

The line here is that capitalism does indeed teach, or as Foucault would say, impose self-discipline and self-responsibility. But these are in turn sanctioned by traditional and community values and are the requirements of a free market which in turn is a generator of prosperity through progress in society.

The key term used by Foucault of, 'otherness' is also particularly questionable. There is no political contrast between madness and normality. Society provides much support in terms of sheltered housing and financial help. Consequently there is still some of the `same' community feeling within the `other.'

This brings together the usual foci on language and attitudes but this is largely based on ignorance, prejudice and fear. If the main problem is ignorance much of this could be easily answered through education. We cannot know what a mental illness is unless we have experienced it ourselves. We cannot know its otherness. But we can all sympathize with fear and unhappiness and this should be enough to dispel stigma

An increasingly important issue today is getting back to work. This is the last barrier to social exclusion. Again this is part of our dignity as much as the freedoms mentioned above. If there is to be true inclusion this question must be addressed.

But how deep is the discrimination here? A disability employment adviser can link people in with employers who are sympathetic to mental illness. If we are excluded from this then I think Foucault might still have a point.

Looking at other areas of prejudice, such as racial discrimination, seems to point to two outcomes. In the Stephen Lawrence enquiry there was a charge of institutional racism. Then again look at the positive influence of Martin Luther King...

Flora MacDonalds book on depression, 'Threads

of Hope', encourages the mentally ill to be optimistic about employment prospects. Stigma is not the end of the story and the social worker should perhaps encourage some more positive attitudes in line with the New Deal for Welfare.

So it seems that we can be more positive about mental health than the anti-psychiatry movement. And in practical terms stigma is not such a major problem. But this does not mean we should totally dismiss Foucault.

In any society where self help is esteemed as in ours then however much we come to sympathize with mental illness those who are too ill to cope might always be secondary in status as compared to those who can.

The resulting attitude seems to be that while being

ON ANTI-PSYCHIATRY

ill is OK we must still look up to those who successfully stand on their own two feet and are self-reliant. Stress is good for you if you can handle it and, "Life is hard", so the comment runs.

At one extreme, coping in wartime is still to be admired and bravery rewarded with a medal and the title of heroism. At the other extreme those who commit suicide raise the most direct emotive challenge to stigma.

Foucault seems to be saying that there is at base an essential conflict between society's attitudes and the experience of madness; and, for me, this amounts to the problem that we know we should be disciplined and responsible but we don't feel that way about it.

What makes me wonder though is, as we come to understand mental health more, are we always going to regard people with illnesses as somehow secondary? I am not sure that this point is so easily exploited by Foucault for this reason.

Against the anti-

To reiterate, I have hinted at an important line of thought, instead of transgressing moral barriers so that the mentally ill might rebel against the morals, on which the market depends, maybe there will be some emotional feeling within what Foucault calls, "the other", which may prevent this outcome? The capitalist society that creates the stigma provides much care and community support, so do we really feel so divided from it?

This we noted then raises another set of questions: is there such a political opposition between otherness and normality? Are the two properly separate or is there still some common ground between the excluded other and society? Maybe instead of talk of otherness they are both the same? We are all products of the same culture and society, though we may be, as Foucault claims, in some conflict with its values.

For Foucault, care in the community seems to me to be a gross misnomer. The community only provides care because of the need to control. This group is thus analytically separate from the society rather than `in' it. So the idea of an inclusive `community' is just a way of masking the fact that one social group imposing its values on another to overcome their alienation.

This is primarily done through the support of the family, and personally I have much support from mine. I have made new long standing friends within the circuit of day centres, sheltered accommodation and hospital. As I am not unhappy with my life so I do not feel the alienation highlighted by Foucault.

Community may be defined as networks of friendship and kinship. The conservative philosopher Roger Scruton has argued family feeling and community life is where the fullest expression of our human nature is to be found. These attachments can still be enjoyed within capitalism despite the attempt by Foucault to target its underlying values.

ON ANTI-PSYCHIATRY

There is all the time evidence to the contrary to suggest that capitalist stigma does make us loose some friends and family when we develop a mental illness. This never happened to me and could this be just a result of ignorance? Much of this is the result of media stigma and this, I believe, can be to some extent overcome by education in schools about mental health, which is now to being done.

Another response - different to Scruton - was that happiness rests not with the community but with the individual. This was also the Thatcherite basis of community care which was formulated in terms of the freedom of the individual: that society can teach self-help to include mentally ill people within capitalism and an increasingly individualistic society.

If that seems a bit abstract then it seems necessary to give a personal example. For me it has always been good to meet new people and I look back on my life before the illness enjoying having gone to university at the age of 18. In doing so I chose to move far from my home area and to study in a new social environment, after which I intended to repeat the whole process again by studying for a doctorate elsewhere. During this time I changed my friends a lot and broadened my horizons by living in the different cultures within the UK.

Here the New Deal for welfare is also crucial to the idea of enjoying life under capitalism. We never know where a job will lead and we may be better off for working. Instead of alienation we might see this as an opportunity and it will certainly allows us the dignity of supporting ourselves or making a living for our families etc.

ON ANTI-PSYCHIATRY

We might even enjoy and take pride in whatever line of work we choose to do.

So either way, organic community or capitalist opportunity can be both important to care for the mentally ill. The trick for my own mental illness is to keep busy and not to be socially isolated. I don't mind exclusion from the wider society so long as I can locally choose my friends from the variety people I meet within the mental health system. Variety is the spice of life!

I can hear objections to all this optimism – what a rosy picture of life this is. The big bad world is just a dog eat dog rat race. It is too stressful and depressing a place to be the solution to alienation. It is better not to be involved. But that just amounts in my view on whether the positives in life outweigh the negatives and as I said I am not unhappy despite my notional exclusion.

Foucault's politics, in the end, amount to a call to change the system on the grounds of mental health. Anyone familiar with my essays will note in contrast that there is a great need to believe in the mental health system and inspire hope. If changing the system is the only answer there is going to be less hope all round.

It only remains for me to quote a few common sense style maxims on why changing the system has not happened. There is the belief that, "It will never change." Then there is the thought, "At least we know this system works", whereas other economic systems are untried or, as the pub talk has it in the case of the USSR, did not work because, "It was against human nature", and so on.

ON ANTI-PSYCHIATRY

At the theoretical level the demand to change the system on grounds of mental health begins to encroach on the writings and defences of rightwing academics – some of which encroaches above. The can of worms that this line of thought opens is huge and complex but not without competent challenges to it, as undertaken by Foucault.

How many mentally ill people actually think about the politics of mental health I am unsure? Maybe they just want their lives back or the illness to go away? Maybe too, this does not involve some grand scheme to change the system, just adaptation to unfavourable life circumstances? The political questions raised by the anti-psychiatrists seem interesting, but you can go on arguing about them endlessly.

Capitalist Maxims

The Victorian values celebrated by Thatcherism and behind the great confinement are beliefs or prejudices and even traditions that underpin capitalism. But can we, if people are going to be reasonable and humane, be optimistic about changing the system? To me there are strong grounds for pessimism here and so there seems to me to be a view that if only things were that simple.

The main reason is that to some these prejudices run so deep in our culture. Changing the 'big bad world' is going to be extremely difficult however noble the motivations. It is possible to be sceptical as the view of many people seems to be that, "Life is just like that," and is, "Certainly not a bowl of cherries."

ON ANTI-PSYCHIATRY

This is something which is particularly evident in that they are such a part of some people's outlook that they get to the point that they form the common sense of everyday opinion. These values seem so self evident to many that we rarely get to the point that we question their authority and origins. They are if you like 'embedded' in the culture.

So often then the issue is never discussed. Having a nervous breakdown means that other people might think of it as a failure to cope and so of being weak. The notion of cracking up under pressure is contrary to the belief in the need to be self-reliant and this stigma certainly put me off asking for help.

Men in particular are supposed to be tough. The prejudice is that, "You should not need any help," and you have to, "Just got to get on with it." Again all this thinking reflects common sense and felt to me to be, "Just ignorance." But for me it would be wrong to dismiss capitalism on this basis as this help is available in many ways today.

Prejudice is also an old word and has been used in theoretical writing. In popular parlance it can mean a kind of negative bias towards something as above but in technical terms it refers to a non-rational but none the less cultural belief. The key issue is over how 'deeply rooted' are these attitudes or prejudices in our culture?

The cultural values reflected in capitalist self-help are the products of a long standing way of life and so are justified by that tradition 'it has always been like this.' The thought to some is expressed by the notion that it has always been this way. People are not going to change their values however good their intentions and they will always be imperfect. That is human nature.

ON ANTI-PSYCHIATRY

Capitalism is rooted in many such beliefs: `Every man for himself' and `the survival of the fittest' together means that it is only the toughest who 'get to the top.' This is the thought that this way of life actually seems to work well where any other way is untried and untested. We 'do not know if another way would work as well', as I have often heard it said about the economic failures of the USSR.

As is often pointed out, criticism of negative attitudes towards mental illness strikes at the heart of such cultural beliefs: at the rough tough `stiff upper lip' required to face life's difficulties and to over come them. This Victorian work ethic of self help and self reliance is ultimately also part of the British character and national identity.

So another phrase often used of prejudice is that it is 'endemic' think again for instance of the problems of eradicating attitudes and beliefs about race? There is the charge, even today, of institutional racism levied by the Stephen Lawrence enquiry. Then there is here too the most often used counter example of the influence of Martin Luther King in history. So some things do improve then despite prejudice.

But again it is the idea that this sort of thing is 'endemic' which is what really interests me about the nature of capitalism. So far I have presented the whole thing as the conservative view of beliefs from which we might draw the conclusion that any change is going to be a gradual incremental process. But here there may be a very big cloud on the horizon for improving the social position of the mentally ill?

ON ANTI-PSYCHIATRY

The twentieth century philosopher Michel Foucault thought that the origin of mental health prejudices where not so much cultural as economic. The idea that, "Life is not a bowl of cherries," so, "Pull yourself together", derives from the capitalist ethic of self reliance and self discipline and its `dog eat dog' way of life, for which you need to be tough. For this writer the only way to get rid of prejudice is to get rid of capitalism.

We may pity those less fortunate than ourselves, for example, but the values we must first promote are primarily those on which the system works. This in the end means that the `sink or swim' style `rat race' is deeply rooted in our values and beliefs for many reasons. The thought is that, "The world is just like that," in addition to the belief that, "It is never going to change." We can have the mental health system in capitalism but it is still for Foucault in essential conflict with that culture.

This raises an obvious question: why does mental health exist at all? Here we saw Foucault's answer is that it prevents the alienation of those who cannot cope from become a source of opposition to the system that creates it. He sees `mental health' as a form of social control of an excluded group. One big problem is the consequence that he cannot recognise or at least must devalue the humanitarian reasons that might remove stigma as genuine motivations.

This then puts the whole issue of the philosophy of the free market, which can be construed so that stigma might be a necessary evil to be weighed against the benefits of capitalism, in a whole new light. Prejudice may be necessary to this society and not without its own political justifications:

especially in terms of material prosperity, as achieved through a capitalist economy, and so may be difficult to 'rid ourselves' of.

Opening up the issues

The Thatcher project of community care embraces a number of key essentials: independence, personal responsibility, discipline, self help and self reliance, greater freedom and choice. Foucault's political strategy in contrast is based on a number of interconnected ideas: dividing practices, a carcereal society, the great confinement, social control, cultural limits, transgression and otherness. I take these ideas to be self explanatory in terms of their ideological complexion.

For Foucault we noted the community does not care but controls so that learning self-help through all the variety of places and ways (including day centres, sheltered housing and workshops, education etc) is merely the extensive apparatus of establishing this control. All the enumerable ways of achieving this about which I have written in this book – from my own experiences - are thus reduced to a very subtle set of techniques of establishing some kind of power and domination.

Where the picture from the point of view of Thatcherism is that community care is a way of empowering the individual for Foucault this is nothing of the kind. Instead of being enabled we are controlled. The power we have is merely the way we become subjected to the ideas and values of capitalism. But if this is true what has become of our freedom?

This question is particularly interesting from the Thatcherite community care angle because the whole point of the policy was about individual freedom. For Foucaultians the liberation from the asylum was nothing of the kind. Rather what happened is a form of confinement was replaced by a new system of control. Social exclusion thus became the excuse for a more effective form of domination called social inclusion?

So if Foucault's 'dividing practices' can in practice be in many ways overcome we are going to have to get into the nitty gritty of service user experiences of social services and caring support to see how far it accords with experiences and perceptions. This of course might provide a tool kit for political resistance or might lead to the outcome that to say the social worker who does the care are at the same time subjugating their clients?

Obviously the most visible expression of diving practices is stigma which may well be difficult to eliminate because as I have argued it is so deeply rooted in beliefs about capitalism and human nature etc. But society does not simply say pull yourself together it provides support to enable people to do so. This as Foucault may perhaps have said was, 'in line with its values?'

The images of dividing practices to my mind seem to conjure up other images that the mentally ill club together because they are socially excluded and that life must still be limited to the confines of the mental health system. Actually for me there is not a new form of confinement here as life within the system is pretty much the same in the many ways I have indicated as life on the 'outside' of it.

Many writers also concentrated on the worse side of the stigma like Goffman who begins with the idea of normality (or normalising in Foucault). Actually many activities available to normal people are available to others. In the end I feel that this is just a word and when we begin to live a normal life the politics of all this can be challenged too.

This for me is not just a way of words since any serious discussion of the politics of mental health in terms of community care will inevitably make use of the ideas to help liberate the mentally ill whether that is from the left and right of the political spectrum. But for me it is the individual feelings which these ideas try to engage with which is the most important thing to deciding the issue.

If a person as in my case is not unhappy with their lives to what extent does their treatment by society influence this? Is it fair to say that my contentment is just a sham because I have been somehow manipulated into a state of wellbeing by my upbringing and the mental health system?

The affirmative answer to all this is that the more we (or at least me) ponder it makes Foucault's comments sound a bit speculative when contrasted with the actual way we feel cared for – that is whether this is by family friends and other forms of support. If this is simply domination then we might forgive those who choose to have what are the most important things in life?

Also what then of the role of carers and people's families? People do and might inevitably care about each other, else why would we care about such domination? I think the account in Foucault's terms makes this into a kind of sham if the only relevance here is that carers too are in the end part of the system of domination and enslaving their friends and relatives. What kind of family would that really be?

ON ANTI-PSYCHIATRY

This suggestion to Foucault would be a huge step too far. It is not a crude theory that society provides care simply to ward off alienation. In fact as we shall see actively enslave ourselves because we are not thinking enough about accepting these contentious values and may not thus be acting in their best interests at all?

But that to me is putting words into my mouth. It assumes that my best interests are not apparent to me, or at least my real interests? It means that capitalism is so repugnant that family life cannot make life within good enough to put up with its negative aspects. These for me must be balance against the value of a free market and what that can do for people (apart from just alienating them).

I now want to put the aspects of family and community life whilst mentally ill in the context of my own writing and experiences. This should hopefully give an example of the sorts of things I am talking about. To do this I have chosen the themes from previous volumes of the Stages of Schizophrenia as examples throughout.

ON ANTI-PSYCHIATRY

Getting A Life

So far then I have presented the issue of alienation in terms of life within the mental health system and one's own life but I feel also that the issue of alienation turns on more than this. As I expressed at the end of part four of this work much depends on having the same opportunities and prospects as any one else in the system. This does not however lead me to think that I must change capitalism to get what I want in life and it is worth reflecting why.

While I do think that capitalism is the only economic system available I am not led to despair at the prospect that it will never change. Rather I am more interested in social inclusion and what that might do for me. Not being tough myself I do feel that getting a job that would keep me happy enough to live comfortably would be difficult but money is not everything. Some people never get what they want and that to me is just a fact of life.

Here then it must be remembered that many benefits are not means tested and they do allow a certain level of comfort. For me this issue is that it depends on how much a person wants in material terms and I am mindful that wanting more all the time just creates unhappiness. This thorny issue in some respects is better to be just swept under the carpet.

The happiest time in my life was of course before the illness but was not bliss even then. Anyone can get depression or schizophrenia no matter what their financial position and it does seem superficial to say that money is the most important thing in life. It does seem important to me to consider the issue none-the-less but not in terms of levels of inequality but at a realistic look at what else life has to offer.

My training is in politics so I am going to address this issue in the remainder of this book with an occasional look at what society ideally has got to offer against the experience of alienation including family, community, material progress and the freedoms of the individual. Because these are ideals it is important to question to what extent they are supported by the facts and even whether some of these things exist today at all.

Life could be worse but I am not going to start comparing myself too much with persons in other countries with less well nations else where in the world. It may be we should count ourselves fortunate that we live in a prosperous, stable and democratic nation. They are many examples of this sort of thinking but it is not an outlook I share. I do not in this respect know how lucky I am.

In doing this I am going to look at the defenders of the systems we do live in noting that it has many opponents who hold out the prospect of a better world. Just because I have schizophrenia does not mean I want to assess the prospect of such a happier world either. Not because this seems utopian but because I want to assess and question why it is I do not feel so alienated in this one.

The consequence is that I am trying to weigh up the good things and the bad things in life including the empirical down side which contrasts with the ideal. Many of the points about the material benefits of capitalism and the emotional benefits of community can be contested. So likewise I have made reference to how these might also challenge my view of the system under which we live.

I have seized on facts and figures and the views of theorists with which I am familiar but this is not meant to be an exhaustive view of how academics see the system under which we live. What I have done is give an account of capitalist society as I see it. Needless to say most of these thinkers have a rosy view of this way of life, but this is balanced by here by some empirical criticism.

I want to begin this outline with a consideration of providing community care which was based on the ideal of individual freedom. We live according to Tony Blair in an increasingly individualistic society. But participation in this picture of society is in many ways questionable as a way of empowering the mentally ill and we seem left with the question in practice of whether it is such a good thing.

My question in parts of this outline will be a personal one therefore. Namely what theories can be brought against the attempt by Foucault to undermine capitalism with an alienating view of the mental health system and where do I stand as a mental health service user? To this effect I have included some earlier material which I think gives an appropriate example.

The rest of this essay then will be to bring together a number of experiential lines of argument from a variety of sources so that they may be collectively deployed against the views of Foucault and the like. This has yet to be done in my knowledge in relation to theoretical writing and so I hope to contribute to the debate on mental health in this way. We shall begin by looking at the free market arguments.

ON ANTI-PSYCHIATRY

The benefits of capitalism.

There is one important question to my mind of whether much of this rosy picture of enjoying capitalism by getting back into employment is altogether real? This is the basis of the New Deal for Welfare but here too we must take the good with the bad to determine what our political attitude to Foucault's alienation from its values really amounts to.

Do we really 'enjoy' work so much? Most careers just turn out to be jobs. Staying in one job too long may be boring, it is better to have some variety. I certainly found this to be true of Sheltered workshops. In the end I think for me this opportunity amounts to the situation highlighted by Francis Bacon: that we work to live we do not live to work.

We noted at the outset of this essay that capitalism generates progressive change and that this might be a factor that influences our thinking in our potential state of alienation by weighing up the good and the bad in our lives.

The Conservative philosopher Michael Oakeshott has argued that we are, "disposed to be adventurous and enterprising a people in love with progress and change and apt to rationalise their affections in terms of 'progress'."

In my view as a mental health patient there is a lot of truth about people who are, to some extent; in love with progress and that this is one of the better sides to life under the free market. I enjoy the advance of home electronics in particular and feel this has helped get me through my illness by allowing me to turn my room into a therapeutic sanctuary.

ON ANTI-PSYCHIATRY

For example progress today is particularly visible in the advancement of science and technology which has many benefits which are economic and social and in these respects the internet can be held up as an example.

I have already noted and in previous essays that I have a vast collection of music, films and games and good equipment to play them on. I could get a car if I wanted and have the freedom to go shopping. I do not envy those better off than myself and spending my time pursuing these and my education interests I rarely get the time to dwell on 'comparing myself to other people.'

So in some ways life under capitalism does progress but this is not without its cost and so computers for example have created much unemployment and consequent social problems. I am conscious that I would not like to live in a 'sink estate.' Living in an inner city is a prospect that alarms me however independent and prepared I might be with the help and support of the mental health system.

We may add to the line of thought we have been pursuing then by looking at the nature of the society as well as the economy. But life under capitalism is not just about getting a job and being part of whatever local community. The most important thing is family life and this of course has attracted much debate as well. The whole area is too complex and detailed but it is instructive to consider a particular case as my own as a way of speaking out.

Life and the mental health system.

ON ANTI-PSYCHIATRY

We have noted much of the critical force of Foucault's argument is derived from the view that the alienation of the mentally ill could be otherwise.

But this is in a nutshell exactly what I also think but mostly my experiences of the mental health system suggest a very different answer, and one which has conservative political implications.

I have stressed in my writing that part of my answer to mental health problems have been to spend more time with my new friends and family. Anyone reading my essay above may have assumed that I see life in terms of being born to shop!

This works for me because conversation is distracting and therapeutic and is as effective because it is another form of keeping busy. I do not keep to myself and not being a natural loner find talking interesting and entertaining. Indeed often my conversation is about politics. So I also really enjoy group living and day centers.

But I am also conscious that during my own experience of depression that my family could not cure the symptoms. This was precipitated precisely because of the workings of the capitalist system. When our business went bankrupt we lost our family home and in turn it may have partly caused a relationship break up. My family were there for me but I still felt acutely ill and this feeling lasted for about five years.

Eventually I came round with the help of the mental health system and would now describe my situation as content. Often things are not as bad as they seem. Then again to strike a more optimistic note maybe the future will be better than now?

ON ANTI-PSYCHIATRY

However it may be that the values we impose through stigma may mean we never achieve any such reconciliation with the society because there is such a deep feeling of alienation – most vividly possible in the case of a life long illness. We know we should feel disciplined and responsible but we just don't think of it that way.

This can make the process of upholding existing values very difficult and social influences too are unlikely always to be so 'fulfilling?' The whole situation from Foucault's perspective thus begins to look a bit coercive to some people at this point.

At the end of part four of my book I too expressed some reservations when I was confronted with this prospect of being ill for the rest of my life. Looking at the future I began to ponder if things will never change and whether I would never get to the same position in life which I had when I was 21?

My answer was to simply 'get on with the life I have got' rather than 'dreaming of the one I had' and 'not to waste time doing so.' While I think it is OK to lament such things it is 'better not to dwell on them.'

Thus the recognition for me is that both positions can be very one-sided and are blind to the fact that there may be some truth in both perspectives I have alluded to – those of anti-psychiatry and that of conservatism.

However while my experience is not blind to alienation we noted Foucault seems to me to be blind the existence of such sameness within the other. Foucault attempts to paint the whole world of mental health black.

This seems to me to lead him to discount any thought of compromise or reconciliation as just another attempt to instill discipline, responsibility and the like.

From my experience what this 'alienation' consists is more emotional rather than moral. In this emotional state I can be reconciled by community emotional and family feeling by thinking the issue through.

My view is that Foucault is trying to create the very divides he diagnoses by setting up a series of what to me are just theoretical categories.

The trick when I have felt like this is to 'try and make do with what I have got,' and also to be 'try to be happy with what I have got.'

Part of the answer to these material concerns maybe too it is 'better the devil you know.' Utopian alternatives have often turned out to be dangerous social disasters, with much loss of life. Life under capitalism is not exactly perfect but could be a lot worse under another system of government.

Personally I do not relish the thought of queuing for food under communism and that would certainly make me more depressed. Even if I am less well than some I am mindful there might not be any plausible answer to this. Nevertheless if many readers are like me it is difficult to remind ourselves that we do take much for granted.

At the political level there are of course many other affirmative attachments I feel in life than friends and family.What expresses this is the emotional engagement with politics through the formation of 'attachments' including the 'love of one's country.' We may identify with our way of life and be proud of many English traditions.

This feeling for me has not stopped just because I am schizophrenic and not living in Britain would certainly make me feel much more depressed. That comparison at least does occur to me sometimes.

Family Help.

Family is so important because it is for better or worse such a profound experience. One of the most therapeutic elements it can offer is the feeling of being at home and of feeling a sense of belonging and being wanted. From this bond begins many of the attachments and activities that have helped me through and with my schizophrenia.

Although I have felt depressed during my early illness this could have been a lot worse if they were not 'there for me.' Later in my experience of schizophrenia these feelings of depression have gone and have in many ways I have found family life very supportive.

Often geographical distance is a factor in considering effective family contact, especially if you live and work away from home. Nothing can substitute for being in the same physical space.

My response to my early schizophrenia was that I moved back home from where I studying at University. Face to face contact has been very important in my case and even now I have a video phone at home to enable this contact during crisis periods.

My family did not stigmatise me for being schizophrenic but were instrumental in making me see a doctor and in providing supervised outside contact – every day – for over a year spent in

ON ANTI-PSYCHIATRY

hospital. Nowadays I 'go home' overnight each week for a change of scenery and better food!

At these times I can talk and spend time with my mother, sisters and step dad. We can talk about life in all its aspects and I find this gives me a different perspective on my life within the mental health system.

It provides a valuable reference point to the real world and I do not feel so cut off from the 'normal' aspects of life amongst those who do not have a mental health problem.

Many activities available to such 'normal' people proceed unaltered by my schizophrenia. We go shopping and eating out and all the other things that other normal people do with their families. I find all this highly therapeutic and enjoyable.

This practice of going home is like a mini-holiday and often allows me to study and write more effectively. It is a veritable breath of fresh air, something accentuated by the company and opportunity to go for a walk in the area I grew up in.

The 'sociological functionalists' think that ideally the family is like getting into a warm bath which functions as a support for coping with life's problems and stresses. I would not go that far - as I experience it this overstates the case - but I know I can turn to my family for help in a crisis. At these times home is an alternative to hospital.

At its best, with my schizophrenia, my family support is that of TLC or what people on internet dating agencies call tender loving care. It is perhaps the hardest thing in the world to watch their own child go through all the terror and suffering associated with having a mental illness. The natural response of my family is to try and help.

A particularly poignant example of this was when I was screaming in hospital one night and my family were called to my side. I remember my mother crying at the scene. I think this is the most graphic example of such care I can give.

I think that this has brought my family closer together and adversity can have that effect on a lot of people under such cases. On the other hand I have read a study that showed a lot of relatives act differently to their own when a person is diagnosed.

Often in such times families like friends too will 'show their true colour' though the other possibility is that our 'fair weather friends' will desert us and we will see 'who our true friends are'. But this eventuality is not without its reasons.

I'm not sure that this last point is altogether as bad as it seems even if our friends and family do desert us. This is again because of the pervasive nature of the social stigma surrounding mental health problems like depression and schizophrenia.

The worst case I can imagine is that of a person who might get paranoid about their relatives but that has fortunately never happened to me. Under those circumstances I imagine I would feel very different about any state of alienation.

I guess I am lucky in that I am from a close family and though it has had some problems, notably with divorce, some people are not so fortunate.

ON ANTI-PSYCHIATRY

Family life too is, as we all know, not often all it should be and the kinds of help I am describing are often not available to others.

Family help in the worst cases

In my own case of a failed relationship the experience caused acute depression and my family, friends and keeping busy had no impact on my illness here. Crucially though it would have been worse without them. So I was able to come through it and now think of what happened may have been for the best.

Ironically at my lowest point I was studying and researching Foucault at university and despite his negative perspective on mental health it never occurred to me to think of my own situation politically even though I had acute and prolonged depression.

Nor did I feel alienated from society or other people. I did feel cut off from them because I was not in the same financial position but I had my family and was still not further depressed by these material differences.

I did not feel alienated from these other people however and chose to stay on my course instead of using my qualifications to get whatever kind of job that I could. That may not have been so spectacular but would have made me better off as compared to simply being a 'poor student.'

Some people I know have been abandoned by their families once they begin to develop their mental health problems. In some ways this limits the aspects of fulfilment that I have argued is a political response to the anti-psychiatrists. I imagine too that many patients have been abandoned by their partners and commit suicide.

Single-hood.

It made be argued that a person is not truly fulfilled unless they fall in love and have children and so on. This seems at times to be true but I have answers to even this important criticism as I have explained before.

The prospect of starting a family when a person has a mental illness is a difficult one. Often people with schizophrenia do not get married nor have children. Social Services can take any children a person may have away from them.

The reason is that there is a question mark for many people over whether a mental illness might be genetic and I have read at least one study that if a relative has schizophrenia another stands more chance of developing it. There is a family history of mental illness in my own.

The result of this traumatic thought there is for ones siblings: that once you develop schizophrenia they too may do the same at some point in their life. This may dissuade a person from having children of their own as it would do for me if I was married.

Life without children *is* of course less fulfilling - if not depressing in itself - even where there is close family contact. So too is not being married. However I again feel this outcome without family support would be much worse in my case.

In my case all this has not resulted in the feeling that I am missing out on marriage and children.

ON ANTI-PSYCHIATRY

There are compensations that result from having young nieces and nephews and as I have noted in another essay crucially my affections have naturally transferred to them.

I have had girlfriends within the mental health system and once even being in love. Someone I know who is also about my age has also got married. My feeling about this at present and age thirty one is that it would have to be something pretty wonderful to cause me to do this.

I hope this provides an answer to anyone who reads this looking for a happy ending in my life because they have relatives with schizophrenia that might inspire hope for them. I think it is more hopeful to emphasize the positives I have been describing and say that life can still be fulfilling without this.

It may be thought by many readers that time is running out and for those who are happily married that I am missing out on so much. As I have had one profound experience in a relationship my answer is that I have some idea of what I am missing.

The more sceptical may assume that I have given up hope. But such is life with schizophrenia and what is hopeful is that I can still be on the whole positive about it. I do not feel hopeless so much as having an increasing sense of realism.

Summing up

This essay could have been written in a different way. It could have trawled through conservative defences of the existing social order through the writings of academics against the anti-psychiatry movement.

ON ANTI-PSYCHIATRY

There is a contribution to knowledge to be made here in bringing these ideas together. These are all visible in the works of thinkers who supported the rebirth of capitalism during the 1980's and 1990's and may be deployed against Foucault and the like.

These include the ideas of Roger Scruton who sees community and family as the ultimate forms of human fulfilment. Another is Hayek's link between discipline and responsibility - which we may learn within the family – but which also can be defended as traditional values and as the morals of the free market which generates prosperity and progress.

That has not been my approach however and not because it is not an academic audience that I am trying to reach. Instead I think it is more valuable to suggest and outline how these defences – and positive aspects – of capitalist society as they have come through in my own biographical experiences of mental illness.

In this way I think I can present more of an effective challenge to the anti-psychiatry movement and the thinking of Foucault and Laing, both of whom have never had a mental illness themselves. Only a patient can challenge their thinking in this kind of way.

It maybe that most people have never heard of these writers but they can look them up on the internet and buy their books from Amazon. These writings are academic and I believe it is up to the individual patient to say what they really think of them in practice.

ON ANTI-PSYCHIATRY

As I have said their views seem to paint the whole world of mental health in black but with the right support acute schizophrenia can be manageable and life and while not perfect life within the mental health system can still be at times enjoyable.

We may spend all our time moaning about life or we may try and get on and live it. Whether I will still have the same views ten years from now nobody can predict but I will certainly write a recantation then if I feel the alienation Foucault talks about.

All I can say at the moment after 15 years of illness that I am not in that position. I am now back at university and in part writing about Foucault once again. That will be the moment to make a theoretical challenge to his position - if I pass my exam.

Mark Ellerby

ON ANTI-PSYCHIATRY

Mark Ellerby

ON ANTI-PSYCHIATRY

Mark Ellerby

ON ANTI-PSYCHIATRY

Mark Ellerby

ON ANTI-PSYCHIATRY

Mark Ellerby